Awake, Re and Energized

Making Positive Shifts with the Energetic Well Being Process©

LeRoy Malouf

Merrimack Media

Boston, Massachusetts

Awake, Refreshed and Energized

Copyright 2016 LeRoy Malouf

Library of Congress Control Number:
ISBN: ebook: 978-1-945756-11-5
ISBN: print: 978-1-945756-10-8

Published by Merrimack Media, Boston, Massachusetts
September 2016

CONTENTS

DISCLAIMER

This e-book, its contents, the self-development approaches that are included, the energetic clearing work done by LeRoy Malouf, the Energetic Well Being Process© (EWBP©), and other energetic methods are in no way intended as a replacement for any treatment by a licensed health care provider. No claims are made with the use of these processes. They are not for treatment or cures of your conditions, symptoms, injuries, illnesses, or diseases. Consult your physician, therapist, or counselor for diagnosis and treatment.

Additional information about LeRoy Malouf and about the Energetic Well Being process is contained in his book, *Knowing and Living your Purpose.*

Energetic Well Being also offers demonstrations, workshops, and webinars (Essentials©, Proficiency©, Advanced© and Positive Power of Being Neutral©). For more information, please visit our website at www.ewbp.com.

Energetic Well Being, Energetic Well Being Process, EWB, and EWBP are used interchangeably throughout this e-book.

FOREWORD

It is my pleasure to introduce LeRoy Malouf and his latest work—a treasure chest filled to the brim with insightful information that will inspire you to live in a natural state of wellness, vitality, energy, peace, calm, clarity, love, joy, satisfaction, productivity, and kindness!

Since meeting LeRoy in 2009, we have worked together to inspire and support each other. Eventually, this led to us hosting a seminar together in Egypt. I love to share a funny story about LeRoy, because it exemplifies his wonderful sense of humor and youthful exuberance for life!

I had arrived in Egypt earlier than him and had arranged a tour of the Giza Pyramids for noon, because LeRoy's flight did not arrive until the wee hours that morning. When I informed our guide, "LeRoy is 80 now and it is a long flight. He may want to sleep in," she asked if he would require a walker. I giggled and replied, "No, that will not be necessary." Shortly after, I received an impatient phone call from LeRoy at 9 AM, asking, "Where are you?! I have gone for my swim and answered my emails. I am in the lobby waiting for you to go for breakfast! When do we leave for the pyramids?" That afternoon, we made the long climb up the pyramid in 42-degree Celsius heat, and upon reaching the King's

Chamber, I whispered under my breath, "Act old." I still chuckle whenever I think about his incredulous expression, "What do you mean?" I explained, "It is busy! Act like you are old and need to rest. I want to have time to sit in the energy!" "Oh! OK, I get it!" he replied and accommodated me. This led to a unique opportunity for each of us to lie in the sarcophagus and absorb that powerful energy, one of many beautiful encounters that I have shared with him.

LeRoy walks his talk! After a powerful spiritual experience in college, he made a conscious decision to be in the flow of joy, peace, and love and has stayed true to himself, leading the way with full confidence to inspire self-reliance in others. He empowers people to remember their true potential and create strong internal support for their desired state of being and for what they want in their life. As founder, developer, and owner of Energetic Well Being Process (EWBP) and the Essentials, Proficiency and Advanced Workshops, Home Study Programs and Webinars, and author of *Knowing and Living Your Purpose*, he expertly combines his skills as an applied behavioral scientist with his wealth of knowledge and years of experience in living and loving a full life, not only in his work but also with his family and in his 63-year marriage to his sweetheart, Toni.

I have personally experienced the powerful effect of LeRoy's work in my own life and in the lives of many people at demonstrations, seminars, and as a regular guest on my radio show, *The Truth Is Funny, shift happens* . . . where he expertly and positively shifts a caller's challenging situation at warp speed! His focus is to remove the cause of symptoms rather than alleviating or suppressing them or "learning to live with them," allowing you to live in a continuous state of transformation, rejuvenation, and regeneration.

These pages capture LeRoy's true essence as he brilliantly takes complicated subjects and chisels away to reveal simple concepts that are easily understood and effortlessly applied. As you advance through the book, you can literally feel every cell and process in your body dance in *cell-e-bration* as you renew and rebirth possibilities in every area of your life: physical, mental, emotional, psychological, psychic, and spiritual.

—Colette Marie Stefan

ACKNOWLEDGMENTS

I feel very blessed by, and am grateful for:

The Certified Energetic Well Being Process© Practitioners and Instructors, and numerous clients and colleagues from all over the world who have trusted, shared with and taught me over the last several decades.

The great Foreword by Colette Marie Stefan, who is a magical speaker, author, and artist with a great sense of humor who shares universal, life-transforming information to provide results that will inspire you to soar with her to new heights at seminars around the globe.

Five Certified Practitioners and Instructors have been particularly active in supporting the broader exposure, understanding, use, education, skill and delivery of EWBP – Selina Denny, Chuck Goodwin, Karuna Joy, Adam Khedoori, and Gary Niki!

Selina has amazing and wonderful skills in communicating with the spirit world, and in supporting the expansion of spiritual awareness. She is an inspiration to me, which has enabled me to increase what I do in helping and enabling others to increase their spiritual awareness, and in making positive shifts for all living things, and for the universe as a whole.

Chuck has been conducting monthly support group

calls for those who have attended at least one workshop, and has eagerly worked with new practitioners to help them increase their capabilities.

Karuna has been teaching new participants in how to understand and use EWBP to help others.

Adam and I have worked intensely to re-design and repackage the "Positive Power of Being Neutral Workshop" as an online course available at Udemy.com. If a coupon is obtained at ewbp.com participants get a big (currently 50%) discount.

Gary has been present at every Free Demo and workshop that I have conducted in the D.C area over the past 2-3 years, and has assisted in the set-up, understanding, facilitation, and delivery of these events.

Dr. Margaret Gennaro, who does amazing work bringing wellness and vitality to numerous patients, for her support over many years, and for her review of the impact of this work on two of her clients she referred to me.

The many who have hosted free EWB demonstrations and workshops.

My current Office Manager, Heidi Hudson Bassett, and many wonderful others, who have supported me and made it possible to do this work.

Over 63 years of marriage with my wonderful, loving wife, Toni.

Our family of six children, twelve grandchildren, and six great-grandchildren.

Having high energy and vitality almost every day, and for the intuition and insight to communicate with ascended guides, masters and teachers, councils, boards, and angels.

Living and working in a great location, Cape Cod, Massachusetts.

Contact information for all of the above is available at ewbp.com.

LeRoy Malouf

INTRODUCTION

All too frequently we find ourselves "stuck" with one or more issues or challenges, such as physical, mental, emotional, psychological, spiritual, financial, or relationship. We may try many ways to deal with them, some without success. We have difficulty getting back to our natural state of wellness and vitality. We don't realize that many of our patterns of living in the world are actually causing our energy to weaken, and that we are creating our own symptoms. Mostly, we just want to be free of our symptoms so we can get on with our lives. We work at it, but the symptoms often don't go away and may keep getting worse.

The good news about us human beings is that we are very creative and complex. The bad news about us human beings is the same thing! It is often a challenge to figure out what is going on with us, what is bothering us, and how to deal with it. Learning to do so is a skill-building process to help us deal with all of this complexity and figure out how to clear away our symptoms and create support for what we want in a straightforward way. This e-book is an introduction and overview of how the Energetic Well Being Process© helps to create these skills.

The Energetic Well Being Process© (EWBP©) is an energy modality focusing on quickly clearing away our symptoms and getting us back to our natural state. EWBP uncovers the intelligence behind symptoms, pointing toward life issues that are root causes of what we are experiencing. EWBP then enables us to delete the symptoms by clearing the root causes.

I want to explain why I structured this book in the format it is in, using the brain as an example. We often describe the physical structure of our brain as being the left brain and the right brain. Our attempts to describe how these two hemispheres function are less precise. A way of doing so is to describe how we process information and how we go about functioning.

For example, we talk about the function of the left hemisphere as being rational, thinking, and processing information in a linear step-by-step manner. The function of the right hemisphere is described as being creative, connected with our emotions, and multidimensional as compared to linear.

Most courses in our schools are structured to teach us through the left hemisphere. For example, think of learning history by learning dates, events, who was involved, their roles, and how they impacted others and history. This is mostly left hemisphere, rational.

Others are structured to help us learn through the right hemisphere, or through both. Another way of teaching history is to pick a major event, present all of the historical documents that describe what was written at the time by those who were strongly supporting a major decision that was made, and the documents that were written by those who strongly supported an opposite decision. Then, ask and guide the students to think about how to analyze and understand the situation from both perspectives, and to come to a conclusion about what they would have done at the time. This is a way to teach using the processes of both hemispheres.

A third way of teaching history is to tell stories. We get insights by listening to good storytellers. We hear about how wisdom and understanding of a tribe or nation is passed on through oral traditions. For example, there is a story about how my ancestors had to move the whole population from one location to another because they were in the path of an approaching marauding, slash and burn, large army that they had no hope of defeating.

At first glance, this e-book may look like it should have been two books, because the first part is more of a left-brain description of how EWB is structured to help us eliminate our symptoms and create support for our desired states. It includes specific steps you can take to keep bettering yourself, as well as four client examples, which are stories of success to illustrate the efficacy of the Process.

This part gets us to *stretch forward* both by helping us to experience how quickly our symptoms can be removed, and thus to shift our mindsets and assumptions *from* believing we have to struggle through this life *to* believing we are able to live a life of ease, flow, and joy. It also helps us make this shift by remembering times in our lives when we have experienced unconditional love, which ends up being a great and necessary way to deal with the anger that most of us are carrying. Our experiences and feelings of unconditional love is the best description there is of who we really are. This helps us keep figuring out how best to live our lives, and to get stronger and stronger to more of our lives.

The second part is made up of conversations with spiritual beings, ascended masters, angels, teachers, and guides. This is more of a right-brain approach to help us remember more about who we really are, and thereby to be stronger and more fit in all ways as we live our lives. It uses these spiritual discussions to *pull us forward* by revealing insights to inspire us to live in more joy and peace.

My wish is for this book to help you, the reader, to find ways to be stronger and more fit in all ways as you progress through this life! A way to measure what is meant by "being stronger and more fit" is to respond to this question –

What % of your days do you "Awake, Refreshed and Energized"? When I ask people this they say "Yes, that's what I want to do!"

And…the average for us human beings is "around 20%". Where does this number come from? There is a description in Chapter 1 of the % of our lives we go strong to, and it averages about 20% for adults. Which means our energy is going weak to about 80% of our lives! Hard to believe? Think about how much of your day involves upset, reaction, judging yourself and others, creating drama, being depressed, focused on what is bothering you, being bothered by a relationship(s), etc.

As the proverbial lawyer says "I rest my case"! Read on and apply, and you'll more likely 'awake on the right side of the bed'!

CHAPTER 1.

HOW WE CREATE OUR ISSUES AND SYMPTOMS AND DEAL WITH THEM

Have you ever felt or heard, "I have this symptom (pain, migraine headache, depression, acid stomach, sadness, cancer), and I've been to many traditional and alternative practitioners/modalities, and it won't go away"?

To get a deeper understanding of why our symptoms persist or get worse, and how they can go away quickly, I find it helpful to understand how and why we create symptoms. How do we move away from our natural place of wellness, vitality, and knowing and being who we really are?

It appears that one of the biggest paradoxes about human beings is that *we don't support what we say we want, and we don't let go of what we say we don't want.*

One experience I've heard to illustrate the above paradox happens in January, when people enthusiastically join a gym with the intention of working out regularly. There are numerous people in the gym the first week. The third week only about half of them show up. By the first week in February, there are very few new people showing up.

When you ask people how often New Year's resolutions

become reality, there is usually a laugh and then the response, "Almost never!" So what is going on? This is a quandary, since we truly do want to keep improving ourselves and living better lives.

My favorite way of explaining what is happening is to contrast the lives of five-year-old children with the lives of adults. It is widely observed and quoted that they laugh 300–500 times a day! And, that the average adult laughs only 5–20 times a day. I have observed in others and myself that on a "bad day" we have trouble laughing even once. The children are going strong to 90 percent of their lives, and the adult to 20 percent.

Children live primarily with positive or expanding patterns, thoughts/beliefs that create strength, wellness, and vitality, such as:

Thoughts and emotions: Self-love, self-acceptance, forgiving ourselves and others, patience, kindness, generosity, gentleness, gratitude, harmony.

Beliefs: "I am enough." "People mean well." "People look out for and support others." "This is for my greatest and highest good."

Assumptions: "My family loves me." "My coworkers have my back." "Money flows naturally." "It all works out just fine."

Desires: "To know and live my purpose." "To make a contribution in the world." "To care for and provide for myself and my family."

A big shift takes place as children are taught and told how to "live in the real world." Unfortunately, what we as children are taught often does not support our wellness and vitality (consciously and unconsciously). We spend much more time and effort thinking our way into problems, symptoms, or situations without being aware of it. Part of it is that we are not mindful of the negative implications of our negative thinking. We don't realize there are short- and long-term consequences.

We are taught numerous negative or limiting patterns, thoughts/beliefs that create weakness in us, such as:

Thoughts and emotions: Self-judgment, judging others, ongoing anger, resentment, inferiority, superiority, guilt, fears, and other self-deprecating thoughts and feelings.

Beliefs: "You can't find people who want to do good work." "There are no quality products anymore." "You have to do it yourself." "People (who don't think like me) are stupid." "Drivers don't care about anyone else."

Assumptions: "There's no sense placing the ad, no one will respond." "You can't teach an old dog new tricks." "My friend is always late." "There is only so much one person can do." "I can't do that anymore."

Limitations: Retreating behind excuses of helplessness, holding on to the past and to ways that used to work.

Desires: "I need/must have/crave money, sex, a fix, control, company, good looks, respect, adulation, etc."

There are many ways like these that we block ourselves. We create, buy into, and take on these blocks from our ancestors, our parents and relatives, the people we socialize with, work, peer groups, our experiences, our environment, society in general, and so on. These blocks become patterns that are "normal" ways for us to think and act. These beliefs and messages play in the background of our thoughts, minds, and bodies.

Any one of these ways of weakening our energy is small, but when we accumulate many of them over days, weeks, months, and a lifetime, we get energetic blocks. We block ourselves physically, mentally, emotionally, psychologically, physically, and spiritually.

Eventually we say, "Ouch!" when such inner messages

manifest into symptoms, a disorder, or disease. They are indications of some disharmony within ourselves.

HOW WE NORMALLY DEAL WITH SYMPTOMS

Our conscious and normal approach is to try to get rid of or reduce the symptoms instead of eliminating the root cause(s). We:

- Take over-the-counter remedies, supplements, herbs to reduce pains and other symptoms.

- Take prescription drugs to reduce symptoms and to get our bodies to function better.

- Take more drugs to deal with the side effects from the drugs we are already taking.

- Use some form of stress reduction to feel better.

- Get operations to cut out some offending parts of our bodies.

- Participate in numerous modalities and treatments.

- "Cope" and learn to live with the symptoms.

- Suppress the symptoms by forcing ourselves not to think about them.

Fortunately, there are numerous traditional and alternative approaches, treatments, products, and modalities for helping people. And, fortunately, they work for numerous people! Most of these are helpful and the symptoms often go away. However, nothing seems to work for everyone. All too frequently, people say they have used many modalities and:

- Their symptoms are not going away.

- They go away for a while and then come back.
- Additional or worse symptoms show up!

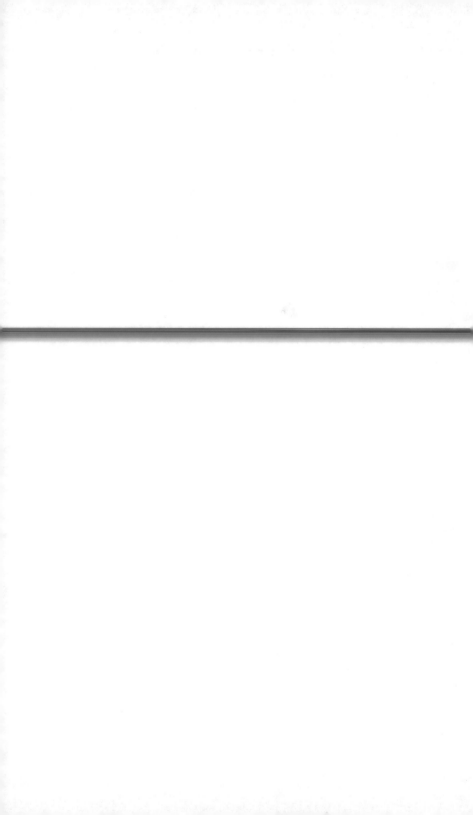

CHAPTER 2.

HOW TO MORE EFFECTIVELY ELIMINATE OUR SYMPTOMS

Let's look first at what is broadly accepted as working with energy: "Energy medicine, energy therapy, energy healing, or spiritual healing is a branch of complementary and alternative medicine based on the understanding that a healer can channel healing energy into the person seeking help by different methods: hands-on, hands-off, and distant (or absent), where the patient and healer are in different locations." (Wikipedia)

A key belief on which energy work is based is that we want to be well and fit, in spite of the many ways we actually cause our energies to go weak. We want to live in wellness and vitality as a normal part of everyday life. We observe that our bodies and spirits are designed and constructed to support us being in a healthy state. For example, we get a cut and it heals. Or, we are diagnosed with a disease and our body eliminates it and becomes stronger in repelling the disease. Our immune response is flexible and is usually quite capable of dealing with agents that threaten our physical wellness.

Our bodies continuously (every second) create 15-20

trillion new cells to replace dead or diseased cells, or those that are not functioning well.

We get unhappy or down about something to do with ourselves or in a challenging situation, draw our energy in, then get an insight or idea about how to move ahead. Then we turn it around and move forward with positive intent and excitement.

THE ENERGETIC WELL BEING PROCESS© (EWBP©)

I call the way I work the "Energetic Well Being Process." EWBP works with a person's energy to clear away the blocks we have created and bring about wellness. EWBP transcends traditional and most alternative approaches. It is an energy strengthening modality that is based on what I have learned from:

- Other modalities (Agnes Sanford's, "Healing of the Soul"; Yuen Method; Theta Healing; Matrix Energetics; EFT; Keith Varnum)

- Spiritual experiences (Baptism of the Holy Spirit; Prophecy; Speaking in and interpretation of other languages; Spiritual Healing; Casting out of Demons)

- Instruction and guidance from ascended masters and teachers (Jesus, angels, archangels, spiritual councils, and others from this and other universes)

- Insights from my work with myself and with clients that results in ways to clear problems, in protocols that I have not seen or heard of before, and in discovering new ways when working with other practitioners.

In its simplest form, EWBP helps clients strengthen their energy and discover their truth, and that truth sets them free. Their symptoms go away and they regain their natural state of wellness and vitality. This is so simple that clients often have difficulty understanding it.

A way of illustrating this comes from what we learned from quantum physics — that the act of observing a quantum particle causes it to change from a particle to a wave. Observing a wave causes it to change to a particle. The parallel here is that when you connect a person's symptom (of pain or depression) to the truth of the life issue(s) that is the root cause, the act of observing the truth deletes the root cause. The symptom clears away. It's as simple as that!

Understandably, we want to get rid of the symptoms so we can feel better again. Another way of thinking about this is that symptoms are signals to us, a way of communicating with ourselves. They are signals about what is causing us difficulty and that we need to do something about it! These symptoms are saying, "Hello, I know you're very busy now, but there's something out of order that you need to take care of."

What happens when we don't remove the symptoms? Our inner self turns up the "volume" and the symptoms get worse! They are saying, "Can you hear me yet? You really do need to take care of this!"

Note that a *key assumption* on which most of the normal approaches referenced to in Chapter 1 are based on is that a very high percentage of the root causes for our symptoms are *physical*. Examples are:

"My neck pain was caused by whiplash from a car accident."

"My back is hurting because I slept wrong or I lifted something the wrong way."

"I got a cold because there was a cold breeze blowing over my head while I slept."

"I was not watching what I was doing, I stubbed my toe and I could barely walk."

With the approaches that many people take to deal with these symptoms, some key questions to ask are: *Were the symptoms completely cleared? Do they come back? Do we have to keep struggling with them?*

One good lesson I remember from my mechanical engineering training is that, "If something is not working, turn it around and approach it from the opposite direction." What if we approach symptoms in the same way? What if the root causes for the symptoms have *non-physical* causes instead of physical causes?

CHAPTER 3.

OUR SYMPTOMS HAVE INTELLIGENCE

If our natural state of "being" is wellness, why wouldn't we give ourselves clues as to how to get back to that state? What if our symptoms are trying to get us back to living our lives in our natural state of joy, wellness, and vitality?

Suppose we changed our view of symptoms. Instead of thinking of symptoms as bad and something we have to get rid of, what if we think of them as only energy, neither right nor wrong, nor good or bad? (At first, we may have a lot of trouble believing this, especially when we are feeling really sick!)

What if the symptoms are signals trying to guide us back to wellness? What if they are messages from our wise inner-selves to our conscious mind to enhance our wellbeing? This may be a bit of a stretch if it is a new idea to you.

Let's consider how all of this looks from the assumptions that:

The vast majority of the root causes of our symptoms are non-physical. They are predominantly *life* issues. Anything and everything in our life that bothers us causes our energy to go weak. What bothers us the most? Issues we have with money, relationships, health, control, work, etc.

Our symptoms have intelligence and are pointing us to the life issues that are the root causes. It probably sounds odd to refer to our symptoms as having physical intelligence. Generally, what most people want most is just to get rid of them. What if the symptoms actually contain clues about what we need to deal with in our lives that is bothering us and creating the symptoms and illnesses? Remember, our energy goes weak in response to everything that is bothering us.

HOW TO INTERPRET WHAT OUR SYMPTOMS ARE "TELLING" US

The locations of the symptoms are frequently direct indications of underlying roots:

A client named "Terri" (assumed name) complained of a pain in the neck. When asked, "Who or what in your life is a pain in the neck?" she said, "Oh yeah, 50 percent of my job is boring, my husband expects me to be his waitress, we're always short of money, we're receiving frequent unwanted calls from telemarketers," and so on, for a total of seven things bothering her.

The key to unlocking her constant pain that she had for 25 years since she experienced whiplash in an auto accident was the question suggested by the pain-in-her-neck symptom: "Who or what in your life is a pain in the neck?"

It took forty minutes to help Terri find the seven major things in her life that were bothering her, and her pain completely went away. It was finding her truth that set her free!

Twenty-five years of believing what was not actually her truth ("the whiplash caused my neck pain") actually perpetuated her symptom. The many options she pursued for eliminating her pain did not work, because the seven contributing issues in her life (or more as time went on) would have persisted in bothering her. She started having much better mornings!

How do you get good at interpreting what the symptoms are saying? This is a skill that I think of as additional sensory perception. To help improve this skill, we need to keep asking the question, "What are the "life issues" that are causing a symptom?" It helps to practice this skill every day by paying attention to what is going on in your body.

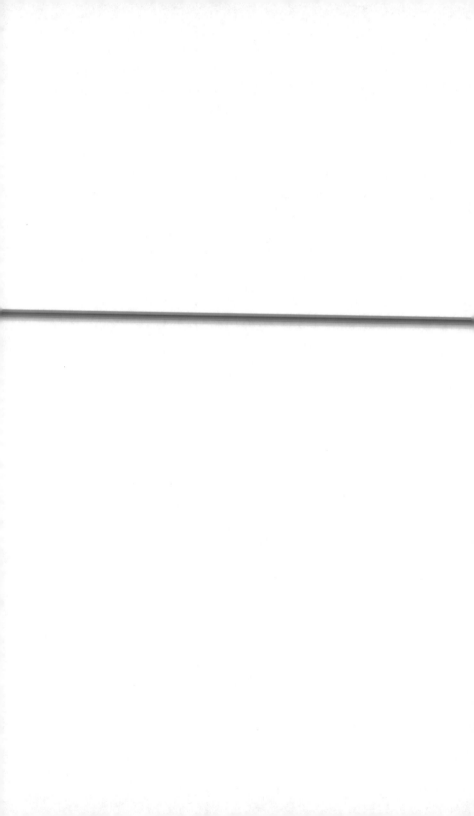

CHAPTER 4.

FOUR CASE EXAMPLES

With a Doctor's Report on the Third and Fourth

Here are four examples of interpreting what the symptoms are saying. In these examples, all of the client work was done on the phone. (First and last initials and disguised first names are used in place of real names in order to protect privacy.)

FIRST EXAMPLE - NOT SLEEPING AND FEELING VULNERABLE

1. H. had been having difficulty sleeping for seven months. What happened illustrates the need to keep searching for the relevant life issues that are the root causes for our symptoms. She described feeling vulnerable or not protected. She related several ways she felt her spouse was not supporting her. I suggested that vulnerability can also be related to where a person is living, but she could not think of anything like that. However, a few days later an email came.

"You asked me what was going on in my area that might be adding to my "feeling vulnerable." I don't know how it escaped me, but yes, a fever has become an epidemic . . . and my husband was one of the first to get it.

"About three weeks before he became ill we got mites in our house. He came down with the fever. It was a very bad case of it. He was given twenty-four hours to get his platelet levels up or else he would be hospitalized. Thank God I discovered what would cure this, and he recovered. During this crisis, we also euthanized a dog (I was giving simultaneous dog end-of-life care and husband save-his-life care), and another dog was poisoned and rushed to the hospital.

"So, yes, there is something going on that leaves me feeling vulnerable!"

This was the key life issue, in its several manifestations, that unlocked the sleeplessness. She is since sleeping well.

Our tendency is to want to forget or suppress challenging or traumatic situations. Yet they can be the direct life issues that are the key root causes. Feeling vulnerable can come from situations such as bullying, abuse, gang or drug violence, house break-ins, loss of money or investments, and so on. Now, contrast these root causes with what we normally hear are the causes for difficulties sleeping: staying up too late too many nights in a row; feeling it is something I ate; eating too late at night; feeling jet lag; experiencing disruption of normal patterns; hearing noise from traffic or neighbors, and countless other such reasons.

Yes, these can cause sleep issues. However, when the sleep issues persist over a long time, it is more likely life issues that are the primary root causes.

Let's examine another example where the location of the symptom was a key in finding and clearing it.

"I'm terrified about a lump in my breast," M.B. called to say. "While doing a self-examination, I found a fast-growing, large marble-sized lump in my left breast. It was hard and growing larger. My doctor sent me to get a mammogram. Upon examining me, the technician and the radiologist made gestures and comments that scared me."

I did a clearing session with her that was focused on eliminating the root causes of the lump. She was upset and scared. We had another session before the mammogram, and a third one afterward. The sessions lasted thirty minutes to one hour each time. As a result of the first two sessions, the lump softened and was slightly reduced in size. I was puzzled that it was not going away, and started thinking about why the lump would be in the breast.

What do breasts represent? There is the obvious sexual overemphasis on breasts and their size, by both men and women, that could probably take several books to examine.

Two main meanings came from looking at the definition of breasts in a dictionary:

Mammary glands—Female mammalian glands that are modified to secrete milk, are situated ventrally in pairs, and usually terminate in a nipple. The definition also included the "emotional mothering and nurturing function of the breasts."

In our sessions, M.B. had spoken of a son she was very concerned about who had been in serious trouble several times. She had strong feelings of protective over-mothering and over-nurturing. She was deeply feeling both. She also had feelings of over-guarding, overprotecting, over-worrying, over-analyzing, and over-internalizing.

After focusing on and speaking this truth, the lump size immediately reduced by 50 percent. There was no time delay – it just shrank! We had two more sessions and the lump was gone and did not return. That was nine years ago and she is completely free of the symptoms. She has no more lumps.

What else was causing the lump? There were other primary areas of non-physical root causes. These came up in two ways. First by paying close attention to what she was saying and feeling. She sounded afraid at the beginning and, especially so, after the mammogram. She was also feeling depressed and unhappy.

Second are the numerous and negative beliefs, experiences, and assumptions in our culture about cancer. There are ways in which these are described (including treatment impacts and side effects, effectiveness of various practitioners and facilities, impact on friends and families, and others that are described in item 2. below). These can have a very negative impact on a person. I have put together a cancer protocol that EWB practitioners use to check to see what are causes for clients' symptoms, which is where some of the following root causes for M.B. came from:

- Feeling fears of degeneration, and of dying and leaving her family: Getting to neutral where there was no "charge" or reaction was key in dealing with these "normal" fears.

- Resonating with negative beliefs about cancer in general and breast cancer in particular: There are numerous levels of negative beliefs in our culture coming from "experts" about environmental and substance risks, low survival rates, and the negative side effects of prescribed treatments. Though M.B. did not have beliefs about having the gene that increases the risk of getting breast cancer, other women may need to clear it. These beliefs tend to create dis-ease. What we pay attention to is what we create.

- Losing sense of joy and happiness: She had unconsciously been losing her sense of happiness for a couple of years. This weakened her sense of wellbeing and immune response.
- Feeling "lumps" in her thinking, such as:
- Thinking that things can't/won't change.
- Feeling fearful of taking the next steps in life.
- Putting everyone else first and not taking care of herself.
- Being bothered by having large breasts (for some clients, it is about having small breasts).

Physical causes accounted for only about 15 percent of the roots. M.B. exercises regularly, eats well, and is in good shape. Both the non-physical and physical root causes were energetically cleared away. The key was in finding the truth of over-mothering and over-nurturing, and the lump immediately shrunk by half. The energy flowing into her breasts was weak. After the fifth session, the lump went away and her energy was once again flowing fully.

Another question is whether these same roots could be causing lumps for other women. A part of the energy work is to prepare for doing the work. This includes being neutral and non-reactive to whatever is going on with a client. It is also important to not assume you know what their symptoms are or what is causing them.

In the normal course of working with clients, a part of the energy work is to check the client to see where their energy is weak and where it is strong.

This experience with M.B. taught me to check clients whose energy to their breasts was weak for over-protective emotions. In energetic checks of over 400 clients with weak energy in their breasts, there have been two or more of the over-protective emotions present in each of them. These emotions create an energy blockage that reduces the normal positive energy flows to breasts (and genitals) in both women and men.

THIRD EXAMPLE – UNRELENTING, DEBILITATING MIGRAINES

Abby reported, "The migraines started in junior high school, around the mid-1960s. I think I dealt with migraines for 45 years (1965 to 2010) before your clearing. Wow! That's a long time to suffer! When Dr. Gennaro contacted you to request you call me, I had been dealing with a constant three- to four-week series of unrelenting, debilitating migraines that occurred one right after the other, and medication wasn't helping.

It took seven sessions to completely clear the migraines. There were many layers of life issues to clear that were key turning points. In many other cases, there is a single key point along with other minor ones. When we started working, Abby was 58 years old, five feet tall, and weighed two hundred pounds.

Abby used to be a dancer and gymnast, and taught music in school grades K-6. She stumbled in class, injured her back, had unsuccessful back surgery, and ended up with fibromyalgia. She still uses a walker while recovering from the physical disabilities.

When I first checked her energy she had pain (on a scale of 10 maximum) of 9-jaw, 9-neck and shoulder, 9-lower back, and 8-migraine. Her mid-line energy was 1 (very low); muscular and cardiovascular exercise strength-2; Depression-10; Dying-9; Joy-2; Living-1; Degeneration-10. She was extremely tired and had a large amount of toxicity in her body. She was stuck in sadness, grief, heaviness, and seriousness.

There were many layers of clearing, including the following: Thirty past lives and 16 generations of ancestors with heaviness, seriousness, sadness, grief, degeneration, weaknesses in body-mind-spirit and numerous other symptoms. I cleared and strengthened weak mid-line and weak nervous, lymph, and elimination systems. I cleared lack of trust and betrayal by her husband and the school system for which she worked.

Abby unconditionally forgave herself, God, four men (including her husband and school administrators), 15 specific women, and women in general. This included clearing a strong emotional feeling that "love hurts." I also cleared for suffering. And all of this was just in the first session!

Further clearings included numerous strong negative emotions, fears, negative religious teachings, and hesitations about getting ready to be well "now." Abby's heavy depression lifted.

Then we cleared the burdens of too many things to deal with, challenges of dealing with the State bureaucracy, feeling she did not have a leg to stand on, several resistances, and numerous ways of feeling hurt. Everything was going slowly in her external life and relationships, which slowed down her metabolism, so we speeded up her bodily processes. Finances, loneliness, and her energy were out of balance, so we also cleared all aspects of her life for balance.

When the vast majority of life issues were cleared away and she became neutral to the others (so there was no "charge" left), the migraine headaches went away.

Abby thanked me profusely. "I no longer see the neurologist (since the fall of 2010), after you cleared the migraines. I also no longer need Pepsi Cola, Butalbital (caffeine), or Imitrex to control the migraines. Halleluiah! My life became immediately easier after the clearing . . . no more exploding head to deal with. I am so grateful I no longer have to deal with migraines, migraine meds, and emergency rooms! I can't thank you enough for changing my life for the better!"

Most mornings Abby wakes up with a smile on her face, and it's still there when you see her during the day! What a great shift!

Comment from Margaret Gennaro, MD, FAAP, NMD, ABIHM

"Abby came to me repeatedly with excruciating migraine headaches from which she had been suffering for 45 years. Nothing was helping. I recommended that she take LeRoy Malouf's course. She also had sessions with him. Not only did the most recent headaches she had for four weeks disappear, but they never returned."

FOURTH EXAMPLE - MISTAKEN IDENTITY

Helena said, "I am 60 years old. At 55 my life was shattered. My husband of 32 years passed.

"He was my life—an international lawyer, Diplomat, and Colonel in the Marine Corps. We had three children, lived in Vienna, Austria, and traveled around the world.

We had parties and went to State functions. This life was over. Now, there was a dining room table filled with papers and I didn't know what to do except cry. My heart was broken. How can I live without him?

"Eventually I went to see my doctor, Dr. Gennaro. She told me about an energy work demonstration in her office. As I sat in the back of the room, LeRoy picked up on my energy. I told him, 'My name is Helena and my husband passed,' and then came the tears. I had been crying for five years. After, I decided to sign up for an EWBP Workshop. I felt anxious and did not know if I could do this or if it would work. LeRoy said that all you have to do is say, 'Apply.' That is what I did: apply!

"Everyone began noticing a shift in me. I felt nothing at first. After the two-day workshop I reached out and started to make phone calls and there was less crying. I felt more alive. I realized I did feel the shift. I worked on myself daily and used the clearing protocols whenever a life issue occurred.

"Yes, EWBP is working and I can do it. At one of the several workshops I attended, I met one of LeRoy's colleagues, who said to me, 'Is your husband dead or alive? You are acting like he is still alive. How long do you want to hold on to this?' They both worked on me to find root causes and to find my true self.

"The primary root issue was that for 32 years, I was living my husband's life and not my own. Once this was cleared, my life changed—all sadness and grief went away like a wave. Now, I was ready to live MY life. I really started to live, taking different classes and doing clearings every day on myself and others.

"I am no longer, 'Helena whose husband passed!' I am a certified Angel messenger on the radio, and have my own business and meet-up group. I am now a Reverend. I feel wonderful, with every day being full of love and joy.

"My purpose is to live MY life, spread love and joy throughout the world, and help other people get to their true self. Thank you, LeRoy, for EWBP, and seeing something I had inside me that I could not see myself."

The key turning point was to clear away a "mistaken identity," an identity that kept Helena in an ongoing state of weakness, sadness, and grief. When she realized that that was not her true identity, all of those symptoms went away, she went back to her natural state of wellness and vitality, and she discovered her true identity.

Imagine how she feels waking up happy instead of crying her eyes out...for years!

Comment from Margaret Gennaro, MD:

"When Helena's husband passed away after battling cancer, she was devastated. She literally would cry almost the entire office visit. Her whole life had centered around him and now she was lost. I suggested she take LeRoy Malouf's course. She also had sessions with him. I am amazed at who she has become. Her confidence and humor radiate as she empowers others with her Angel readings."

CHAPTER 5.

THE FOCUS OF VARIOUS MODALITIES VS. EWBP

The above examples demonstrate that symptoms can be quickly cleared using EWBP. To better understand clearing work, let's examine the focus of various modalities and the EWB Process when working with clients.

Various modalities all have their own areas of focus, for example:

Physical Body – Massage for reducing stress and increasing relaxation; Chiropractic for creating alignment, flexibility, and strength; Traditional and Alternative Conventional Medicine for eliminating, suppressing, and reducing symptoms; and various approaches for detoxing, for freeing up the functioning of the body, and for enhancing the effectiveness of the immune response.

Mental – Various approaches to meditation; self-improvement workshops, for eliminating mental blocks, and for focus and alignment on goals.

Emotional – EFT and the Sedona Method for releasing emotional blocks, and for restoring wellness.

Psychological – Many approaches to Psychology and

Psychotherapy (including Jungian, Freudian, Reality Therapy, etc.) for releasing conscious and non-conscious blocks and enhancing one's presence in the world.

Psychic – Mediums; Angel Readers; Prophecy; Casting Out, for psychic and spiritual wellness.

Spiritual – Religions; Spiritual and Physical Healing for overall wellness.

People don't live and function in just one of these areas of their life. All are interrelated. Different negative patterns interact with each other. And, yes you can make progress by dealing with specific aspects.

The EWB Process focuses on the whole person (physical, mental, emotional, psychological, psychic, and spiritual), clears away blockages in all these aspects, and quickly brings the person back to their natural state of wellness, vitality, and joy.

CHAPTER 6.

SIX KEY COMPONENTS OF EWB

ONE:
DEALING WITH ISSUES WHILE TAKING A LONG-TERM VIEW

Let's put this in a broader context. How do we get ourselves to the place of having many symptoms?

As we discussed earlier, when we are five years old, we are going strong to 90 percent of our life. We are laughing an average of 300–500 times a day. As an average adult, we are going strong to only about 20 percent of our life, and laugh 5–20 times per day. On a bad day we have trouble mustering even one. We know that laughter and fun helps keep our immune response and wellness strong.

We don't keep ourselves in good physical shape. Cardiovascular shape is a measure of physical wellness. Another measure is the structural strength of our body. All of our cells are in a cellular matrix. When it is strong, it supports the physical and energetic functioning of our body. The average adult client is in about 25 percent physical shape.

Reduced physical functioning is reflected by less strength, stamina, flexibility, mobility, and agility, regardless of age.

Reduced energetic functioning is reflected by our reduced ability to deal with our own reactions, upsets, triggers, finances, relationships, and life issues. For example, money is a strong energy, and when our energy is weak we become less able to earn and manage it.

We often don't eat well. Dr. David Perlmutter, a Board Certified Neurologist, describes how we have low gut health, which reduces our immune response, our physical brain health, and our brain functioning. (*Brain Maker*, by Perlmutter and Kristin Loberg, Little Brown and Company, 2015.) The average adult client gut health is 45 percent to 50 percent.

We have low energy in our bodies. The average client energy in the very center of their body is about 50 percent. We need to be at 100 percent in order to live our life to the fullest without feeling too drained or tired.

Seventy percent of clients are feeling and holding onto anger. Anger is the perfect gift because it keeps giving and giving . . . weakness, reactions, upsets, impatience.

As you read in Chapter 1, we tend to get weaker and weaker in our lives due to our many disempowering thoughts and feelings. The weakening effect of any one of them is small. When we accumulate them over days, weeks, years, or a lifetime, we say "ouch" from physical, mental, emotional, and spiritual symptoms.

The following chart illustrates an all-too-familiar pattern in our lives. We struggle along, get symptoms, feel the need to get help and find it, and pretty soon we're back to feeling bothered by our symptoms and seeking help again.

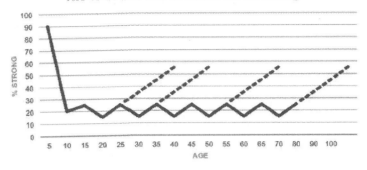

Yes, we need to deal with the immediate symptoms. No one wants to stay in pain or keep struggling with whatever is bothering them.

The difficulty is that as we go through a life of struggle, after we look for and find what helps us to shift and feel better for a while, all too often we encounter more struggle and symptoms! But . . . we have a choice—we can continue as normal, with our energy going weak to 80 percent of our life, dealing with each symptom as it comes along (oftentimes appearing as a crisis), and thus feeling a little better.

Or, we can choose to get back to our natural state of wellness and vitality. How do we make the prolonged positive shift in our life that keeps us getting stronger and stronger to a higher percent of our life, as illustrated by the dashed lines in the above graph? At what point in our life do we make this choice? Generally it's when we hit rock bottom in some way that convinces us to keep improving. For example, a serious illness, accident, addiction, relationship disruption, depression, job or business failure, or loss of a loved one may get us to search for and find ways to shift what we are doing that is not working for us. Or, we may have an experience that awakens us to a positive energy shift that makes us want more.

TWO:

AWAKENING THROUGHOUT OUR LIFE HAPPENS IN DIFFERENT WAYS

Instead of reacting in a crisis, another way of thinking about it is to consciously keep awakening, choosing to stay open and to "keep choosing to BE the real, strong YOU in the moment!" We can keep taking a long-term view by working with ourselves on a regular basis so we are continually improving.

As we stay aware of making ourselves stronger, we can choose any one of the ways our energy is going weak, such as anger, gut health, percentage of our life we're going strong to, etc., and take specific steps to get and feel better in each one.

As we keep making improvements, we are expanding awareness and curiosity, staying open to new possibilities, clarifying where we are and where we are going, trusting, embracing, committing to our passion, accepting transitions, and appreciating our process.

Are there times when this has happened in our lives? It usually happens when we have a significant insight or experience that reveals strong enough benefits to keep us going in a positive-shifting direction. We see or get inspired by some experience, such as a concert, a building project, an athletic event, an art exhibit, a computer program, or a person we admire.

We decide we want to get good at something from which we gain satisfaction, as in playing a musical instrument, learning a trade, preparing for a career, or sharpening a skill in some area of interest. We find a relevant workshop, instructor, coach, guide, instruction book, and away we go.

In the case of a musical instrument, we play our instrument every day. To use this as a parallel, "we" can be the instrument we play every day by continually improving body, mind, and spirit.

Using the EWB Process often helps us to remember who we really are: the True Self, the "I Am" that is one with the Universe.

We get stronger as we get older by increasing our ability to play our instrument—ourselves; and by systematically getting back to our natural state of wellness, vitality, and joy.

THREE:
REMEMBERING THAT UNCONDITIONAL LOVE IS WHO WE REALLY ARE

There are ways for helping us quickly return to our natural state of wellness and vitality. Remember, learning to play a musical instrument or learning a specific skill or sport involves doing it every day in order to increase the necessary skills to excel in it. To apply this to yourself, think of yourself as "me" being "the instrument that I play every day" to be completely proficient at being centered with love in my heart, finding my truth, and living and having fun.

There are many specific steps you can take to keep bettering yourself:

a. Being energetically strong every day.

b. Increasing the percentage of my thoughts, emotions, and experiences that I go strong to with energetic clearing work, and by being neutral to life's events.

c. Increasing my structural strength/integrity with cardiovascular exercise.

...ing grateful for my desired state as though it already
...s.

...owing and building on my strengths.

...ng joyful and having fun every day.

...membering and reinforcing that I am fine in all ways.

...onsciously meditating, being at peace and one with
...ything.

...reasing my gut health.

...conditionally loving, forgiving, and accepting myself
...others.

...continue getting and staying strong, we get into a
...e of Oneness by being strong to "My true self one
...everything, everything one with my true self, one
...divine spirit and order."

...way in which you can increase the positive impact
...our life is to choose which of these steps you are
...kest to and start there by doing what it says. To find
...weakest, ask which of these bothers you the most.
...'s the place to start, which is part of EWBP.

...r example, a high percentage of people (at least
70 percent in my experience) are carrying anger at
themselves or others. If being angry at yourself and others
bother you a lot, then line j. above is a wonderful place
to start because it fuels many different reactions and
judgments!

FOUR:
TAKING A SYSTEMATIC APPROACH TO HAVING THE MOST POSITIVE IMPACT

Step-by-step, the EWB Process of clearing symptoms and
supporting the desired states is:

• Defining the symptom clearly (e.g., my head aches on
the top left side; tension is in my right upper chest; my left
foot is numb).

- Identifying the desired state of being (e.g., my head is clear and feels light; my chest is relaxed and peaceful; my foot is strong, has stamina, is flexible; prosperity; peace; ease). Remember to keep the wording of your desired state in the present tense, not a wish for the future.
  - Clarifying how progress will be measured (e.g., the pain or tension is at level 10 and we want it to go to 0; the person is supporting the desired state at 40 percent and we want it to go to 100 percent).
  - Defining and clearing root causes: Four steps EWBP uses are: (1) finding the truth of the life issues that are the root causes for the symptoms; (2) focusing on full energetic strength in the body; (3) deprogramming the causes (delete them off the brain's "hard drive"); and (4) reprogramming in line with the person's True Self.
  - Frequently checking progress. Continuing until the pain or tension is at 0, and the person fully supports their desired state.

FIVE:
GIVING THANKS AND CELEBRATING

It is wonderful to feel relief when our symptoms are cleared. For example, the pain goes away. What also goes away are any negative emotions from having struggled with the symptoms, such as hopelessness that our symptoms would not go away. It's a time to be consciously grateful!

It's important to be giving thanks for our desired states as though they already exist. The reason for this is that if we keep asking for our desired states, we're acting like we don't have them. For example, if a person's neck pain is cleared by deleting the life issues, and they keep saying, "I wish I'd never had whiplash in that accident," their energy is going weak and they are acting as if the cause for the neck pain still exists. They can actually bring back the pain!

It's also important to keep saying and feeling total neck wellness, which affirms that they are supporting the pain having been deleted. If the pain persists, they need to accept that they have pain (not accepting that they have pain gives the pain energy) but continue affirming wellness. It is not denial to keep affirming wellness even though they may still be experiencing pain. For example, a man in Germany was given a year to live. He kept repeating to himself, "Every little cell in my body is happy! Every little cell in my body is well!" He's completely well, and this can be viewed on www.youtube.com. If a symptom keeps coming back, it is likely that there are other root causes that need to be cleared

Being joyful and having fun are also part of our natural state. There are many times when we experience heaviness and seriousness with our symptoms, which definitely reduces the fun in life. It's wonderful to feel spontaneous joy and happiness again.

SIX:
EXPANDING SPIRITUAL AWARENESS GREATLY ENABLES OUR EXPERIENCES OF UNCONDITIONAL LOVE, AND OUR REMEMBERING AND BEING WHO WE REALLY ARE

There are many ways of awakening, and expanding spiritual awareness is one of these. Different ways work better for different people. Expanding spiritual awareness helps us get to a deeper understanding of who we are and what our purpose in life is. Deeper awareness also helps us get stronger and stronger to a higher percentage of our life. Just as EWBP clears root causes of life symptoms, it also includes expanding spiritual awareness as a way of getting stronger and more fit in all ways as we live our life, and is the subject of Chapter 7.

This is a six-step process for becoming more and more happy in life! And, being happier supports being stronger to life!

CHAPTER 7.

WISDOM ON LOVE AND PRESENCE FROM SPIRITUAL BEINGS

In the course of experiencing other modalities and being open to spiritual growth, I have had the honor of communicating with ascended masters, teachers, councils, angels, and guides. The following is the content of some of these conversations, many of which include a colleague, Selina Denny. The intent is to help increase insights that benefit the reader. There is a heading for the topic of each conversation.

UNCONDITIONAL LOVE

Jesus: I know you have not forgotten me and I certainly have not forgotten either of you. I strongly value our relationship.

LeRoy: Thank you, Jesus. I find your last statement surprisingly wonderful! I normally think of me being like other humans, trying to measure up to even have a relationship with you. I say this even though there are times when you have been demonstrably present, guiding and caring and loving me and others. I'm getting used to us having more frequent and more casual conversations.

Casual is not exactly the word. It's more like very friendly and close conversations. I thank you."

Jesus: I love each of you dearly, as I completely love and accept all humans, all living things, all spiritual beings, and this entire Universe. I also value that you sense the importance of speaking with Mary and Joseph. Please feel free to proceed.

LeRoy: Mother Mary, when I focus on you, I feel this wonderful unconditional love, like I feel with my wife, Toni, and like I, at times, felt with my mother. Thank you for the beauty and presence of the unconditional love that is you! Please tell us what you have for us.

Mary: I very much value the emphasis you have been placing on helping others to be aware of their anger, and of the negative effects it has on them. Also, on helping them to connect with the times in their lives when they have experienced unconditional love, to increase their experience of it, and then to forgive and accept themselves and others. This is one of the very important things you are doing.

Joseph: It is especially important coming from you as a man. Humans often think that this depth of unconditional love is second nature for women and primarily comes through them. As you well know, women can be just as angry as men.

Mary and Joseph: We share unconditional love and acceptance of each other as a model for human couples, as well as for friends to deepen their relationship. The time is coming when this depth of unconditional love will be a bridge for bringing understanding and acceptance between individuals and groups who do not normally think of themselves as being connected through unconditional love and acceptance. As people experience it in more depth in relation to themselves and to their loved ones, they are better able to experience it with others with whom they are not in as close a relationship. We are heartened by your work on Earth, and by the work of so many others who are nurturing and guiding others, teaching them, and being a model of this love.

Selina: Could you please give us information related to the shift from soul presence to awakening? Soul Presence has been important in terms of humans being more aware of and present in their spiritual awareness.

Mary and Joseph: What seemed to LeRoy to be a matter of clarification of Soul Presence indeed was a shift toward understanding that Awakening takes place forever. It happens in different ways with different humans and spiritual beings, and is a way of deepening perception, awareness, understanding, and insight about consciousness, spirit, humanness, manifestation, and presence as times change, and as consciousness increases. Notice how strong your central core is when you focus on awareness!

This also relates to your communication with your Spiritual Council, and other councils, and other beings. It broadens the scope of your awareness and communications! It goes beyond words and thoughts, and increases your understanding of what is being communicated, different ways in which info and intelligence and presence are being communicated, nuances, inferences, and deeper understanding beyond the immediate message.

This is being offered to everyone, and people have different abilities in terms of understanding it, and the invitation to understand comes with assistance from each person's spiritual Guides and Masters.

LeRoy: Thank you. This is fantastic! Do you have any more advice and direction for us regarding our different perceptions or the same perceptions and different approaches?

Mary and Joseph: As has happened so many different times in the past, each of you perceive something from a different perspective and you end up getting mutual understanding, and getting guidance in a way that shows you're working toward the same purpose, even if with different skills and perceptions.

Selina: Humans having to learn from pain and suffering has spiritually ended. Awakening and the coming of Aquarian Consciousness are significant events.

LeRoy: They are not necessarily signaled by a flag going up, or by being loudly announced.

Mary and Joseph: We wish everybody would be more aware of it. Shifts in spiritual awareness often happen with there being one long transition of people becoming aware of greater consciousness, and another long transition out of older patterns. Part of awakening is for people to be more and more aware of what is taking place. If you want, we will set up a fireworks display to make it more demonstrable. Actually, that would probably be welcomed by both of you.

HOLY

LeRoy: I'm seeing and feeling very strong vertical energy this morning, and feeling great peace. Jesus, I hear you saying we need to focus on the word "Holy" in order to deepen our understanding.

Jesus, please help us understand what "Holy" means as the human race moves forward with increased consciousness being available for any and every human. I tend to see that this increase, as described by the coming of Aquarius, is available to everyone, but clearly different cultures and religions will see this in very different ways!!!

Selina: There also is a difference between those who are awakened and those who are in the process of awakening. Those who attended the EWB Advanced Workshop are each in various stages of Awakened.

Jesus: Feel that luminous feeling inside when you focus on holy. Part of the difficulty in your normal human thought patterns is that as the "luminous, holy, magnificent presence" is growing, it is increasingly more difficult to describe in human language as it becomes deeper, more intense, more present than words can convey.

Remember I said that, "By their fruits you shall know them!" That is, as people live love and holiness, it radiates, is infectious, and brings a feeling of lightness, freedom, and awe!

Contrast this living of love and holiness with all the outward conventions, procedures, ways of living and worshiping that humans conceived as what they needed to do in order to be more holy, and to feel like they are living a holy life. These were also ways to show others a direction in which they could become more whole. This is the old way of doing things! It's based on convention and belief and behavior.

The difficulty with this approach is that it sets up a "legalized system" that leads to lots of judgment of self and others, and tends to crowd out the actual presence of love and holiness.

Keep it simple, and get back to, "By their fruits you shall know them, and the fruits of the spirit are love, joy, peace, patience, kindness, goodness, gentleness, faithfulness, self-control." Be at peace!

Selina: In saying that humans are both spirit and nature, and are living very much on this Earth sometimes aware of Earth and nature, and sometimes not, is there a similar list as it relates to the nature aspects of our lives?

Jesus: The parallel that comes to mind is the Scripture to honor thy father and mother! That is to honor nature, care for your environment, be grateful for it, tend it, live in harmony with it, and walk gently and lightly because it completely supports you with all that you need to live this human life! Oh yes, remember to enjoy and be inspired by it, and to see and live joy and peace that is innately nature.

Human beings have evolved from just being able to barely survive, through survival of the fittest, to living in such numbers and comfort, as if they have lost touch with the importance of earth and nature. Both those who are the fittest and those who are not fit have grown in numbers, and are beginning to dominate and override Earth and nature.

Selina: How are we to understand what is happening, and learn once again how to be in harmony with Earth and nature? How do we get back to honoring Earth and nature?

Jesus: Remember that Earth and nature are living systems, just as a human is a living system, and that Earth and nature have symptoms, just like humans get symptoms when they are doing things that cause their energy to go weak. Earth and nature will take care of itself by exhibiting stronger and stronger symptoms (like stronger storms) when they are not being fully supported. That will finally get humans to shift what they are doing to fully take care of Earth and nature!

TERRORISTS AND VIOLENCE

LeRoy: We are faced with fears of more terrorist attacks, with fear the terrorists will get and use nuclear weapons on major cities, and with terrorists who have absolutely no regard for anyone who does not agree with their strict interpretation of Sharia law. They brutally torture and murder those who are not in agreement with them, or are of different faiths, and even those of the Muslim faith who are moderate, and they treat women as though they have no rights.

St. Gabriel: Don't be disheartened by the violence, rudeness, abruptness of others. We stand with you and guide you!

LeRoy: We did some clearing on the Hitler/Nazi era, and are wondering whether or not to apply the same clearing, and what to focus on with the current terrorists.

Would it help to go back to Osama bin Laden and the clearing done then?

St. Gabriel: There has been this violent tendency in humans from the beginning of time. There are humans whose thought processes and motivations focus on murder of others. They are generally called psychopaths. They are in all cultures. Social norms and law enforcement, and fear of punishment generally keeps psychopaths from actually committing murder. It feels like 45 percent of them actually do murder someone. Only about 40 percent of murders are solved, so for many of these psychopaths, it's not a big risk.

The terrorists do not perceive or believe that they have cultural limitations. In fact, the culture that they choose says to actually murder anyone and everyone who is different.

UNCONDITIONAL LOVE AND FORGIVENESS

Mary: It hurts my heart that so many who say they are committed to God and to living their faith have gone so far away from the feminine heart of love in themselves, in their religion, and in their culture. Feel the unconditional love in your hearts, and forgive them for their misinterpretation of the love of God, and for their acts of unkindness, discrimination, torture, violence, and murder.

LeRoy: We ask you to help us to forgive every single one of them, every one of their leaders, everyone who would support them and urge them on, and everyone who would join to commit those barbarous acts.

Mary: It will help at this point for you to feel the

support of all spiritual beings, and of all humans who have love and forgiveness in their heart, and to feel connected by the unconditional love of God. Then, all together to focus on this forgiveness and acceptance. Then breathe in and send it out in all directions to every human and to spread throughout the Universe. As you read this, feel it still working—feel all the hearts joining as one.

Selina: What is the source of this violence in human beings? This sounds like the age-old question of right and wrong, good and evil, selfishness and sharing. The need to be learning from pain and suffering has ended, we don't want it, and we don't want it to come in with the Age of Aquarius!

LeRoy: We are clearing every human being, every past life, every ancestral generation, every cultural belief, every religious belief, every negative embedded thought form, every karmic and traumatic memory and event, and all root causes for everything except unconditional love and acceptance. And I ask all councils, Angels, teachers, and guides to send complete unconditional love, acceptance, and forgiveness to each and everyone from the beginning of time to all human history, past, present, and future. We also clear for all time and space, energies, realities, levels, frequencies, timelines, patterns, universes, dimensions, bodies, and all other negative manifestations, known and unknown.

I'm seeing something like a sunrise, only it's bursting through the middle of the Earth and spreading out to the ends of the Universe and beyond.

We give thanks for being bold and audacious to believe,

in order to pave the way for the full expression and experience of Aquarius. And we give thanks that this is so!

Mary: How is your heart?

LeRoy: Bursting with love and joy! Thank you, thank you! This is what I heard St. Paul describe as the intent of Energetic Well Being.

St. Paul: Notice how the power of the spirit can be so strong and so present and so impactful. When I lived as a human, I felt like I had to walk through all those countries and cities in order to spread the word. Give thanks that spirit has become so much more present in your human hearts so that you can have a bigger impact.

It's time for rejoicing, reflecting, and feeling a greater sense of thanksgiving for all of our wonderful gifts, skills, friends, and unconditional love. That love is still too distant for most people. They've heard of it and sometimes experience it, but still do not appreciate the full power and impact it has had, and that they can have in their lives. The more they are expanding unconditional love in themselves, the more understanding they have, and the more remembering who they really are.

LeRoy: We're calling on all people, angels, teachers, and guides to keep helping those they watch over to expand their knowing, perception, and awareness of unconditional love, to keep awakening, to get that twinkle in their eyes, and to feel gratefulness at a deeper level. So when we focus on gratefulness and unconditional love, these vibrations increase as they spread through and around planet Earth. We're increasing these vibrations and resonances to gain greater entry and oneness with all human beings, and with all living things.

I'm realizing that we tend to think that we can't have such a broad positive impact. And that restrictive thinking, of course, keeps us from doing so. And we're finding out we did have a big impact even when we thought we could not do so.

When there are holidays, the nice thing is that people soften up a bit. They pause from daily tasks. And the shift to celebration is like a portal opening up to help them remember and be more of the unconditional love that they are.

Through such portals we can remember what we were feeling and experiencing with our pets, first love, babies, children playing, enjoying and being one with nature, meditations, spiritual experiences, ahas and deep insights, and deep experiences and relationships, connecting with others and all things.

It can help to capture these feelings in any way that works best for a person, like making a list, and any other way that helps us to recall and expand and deepen our experiences of them.

In a way, they are the best description we have of who we really are: the True Self, Higher Self, Spirit, Divine Blueprint of who we are. Then we take a next step to support all living things.

PEACE

LeRoy: Pastore, could you please give us further information, or definition, and what are we supposed to do about being at peace?

Pastore: I am that I am. I am one with God, Jesus, the Universe. I take the long view, and when I look out through the Universe I see a fantastic energy of love and light that is oneness with the Universe, and yet appears to be spreading. It's like what you see when the sun is rising but just below the horizon, and there's enough haze or moisture in the sky for you to see the rays extending from beyond the immediate view of the sun and yet coming forth and touching everything.

It's time for your work to be coming forth and touching everything. It's actually been happening for some time now already, and you're just starting to appreciate the potentially huge impact that you have. You have this power, and you can and do impact the whole Universe.

Don't shrink back now! Don't buy into the whole belief about how small and insignificant a human being is. That doesn't help you or anybody else. It's time to be bold. You've heard this before and I say it again to bolster your confidence. Don't assume anything about how limited an impact you are having.

I am an angel of God appearing at this time to deepen your understanding of the positive impact of focusing on peace. With all the violence in the world, it's hard to imagine that there can once again be a time of real and lasting peace.

Peace is actually written in your hearts. It is a consequence of, and yet as equally powerful as, unconditional love in your heart. Notice when you say, "unconditional love in your heart," there is huge power and presence. This is the real you. When you do the clearing for increasing your awareness, your knowing, your perception of this unconditional love, you are expanding peace at the same time.

When you then clear to increase your intuition and insight that is based on this unconditional love, and you cleared to get right answers, right actions, right results, and manifestation, you are spreading peace throughout the Universe. In a way, you don't have to look any further!

Yet it seems you want more specific guidance. You are on target to keep posting what you are learning in social media, and finding ways to increase the exposure. You are on target to make this a topic of a radio program. Another option is to write an article about this and publish it. Another option is to put even more emphasis on it in your clearing protocol. And probably the best option is to keep being grateful for the peace that you have and that you keep spreading to others.

LeRoy: Please tell us, when was there a time of lasting peace?

Pastore: There have been numerous times and places all over planet Earth, and some have lasted for a long time and some for only a short time. There is the time during World War I when opposing armies put down their arms and walked across the lines and celebrated. That event brought peace to the hearts of many for many years, and still does when people hear about it. There is the lasting peace that happens with numerous humans when they focus on this place in their hearts. For many, it lasts for most of a lifetime. There are times in many countries when peace lasts for a long time. These may not seem like very much when you notice and realize there are numerous wars and individual acts of violence. Don't let these mislead you into thinking that there is no lasting peace.

CHAPTER 8.

SUMMARY

The biggest paradox about us human beings is that we don't support what we say we want, and we don't let go of what we say we don't want.

We go from being strong to 90 percent of our lives down to 20 percent. Our energy goes weak to everything that bothers us, no matter how big or how small it is. Any one of the times we cause our energy to go weak has a relatively small impact on us. However, when you accumulate it over days, weeks, months, a lifetime, we get energy blocks. We say "ouch" when we get symptoms, whether they are physical, mental, emotional, psychological, psychic, or spiritual.

Traditional approaches to dealing with them tend to focus on their having physical causes, and to reduce or learn to suppress and live with them. It works for many people, but the difficulty is that there are often many negative side effects that also cause symptoms.

There are many modalities that focus on helping people get better and feel well. And, they help numerous people.

The Energetic Well Being Process not only focuses on eliminating the root causes, it also focuses on us continually getting stronger and more fit in all ways as we go through life. The alternative to getting yourself stronger every day is to live with your energy staying weak to 80 percent of your life and creating more and more symptoms for yourself.

A big bonus we get from being consciously strong every day is that it helps us be more aware of how and when we are causing our energy to go weak. When we realize this, we can decide to make our energy strong instead by using options for how to do so as described above.

We can become even stronger by expanding our spiritual awareness. Then we return to our natural state of wellness, vitality, and strength, and with a passion for fulfilling our purpose in life. Thus, we are much more likely to "Awake, Refreshed and Energized"! We may even find that it happens automatically, without our thinking about it!

ABOUT THE AUTHOR

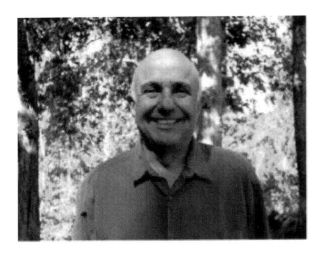

LeRoy Malouf is a strong and fit 84 years young, a wellness and vitality practitioner and instructor, enabling clients to do the same and to make significant breakthroughs and sustainable improvements in their lives. He is the developer of Energetic Well Being Process© and Positive Power of Being Neutral© modalities.

LeRoy is certified in many modalities, alternative healing methods, and consulting and training programs as a multidisciplinary consultant, including being a practitioner of Matrix Energetics©, Ho'oponopono©, as well as being a practitioner and former instructor of the

Yuen Method©. He is also an ordained minister through the Universal Brotherhood Movement.

LeRoy earned a BS in Mechanical Engineering and an MS in Managerial Behavior from the Massachusetts Institute of Technology.

He earned his wings as a pilot, graduated at the top of his training class in academics and flying skill in the USAF, and was awarded a Commendation Medal for outstanding engineering project management. Over the years he has worked with several large organizations and trained and consulted on individual and organizational development. He has been a consultant, Personal, Life and Business Coach and Instructor since 1961.

He founded LMA in 1975, and its subsidiary, SMS, a management and leadership company serving Fortune 500 clients, and worked alongside his children until 2000, to provide consulting services and high-impact training to hundreds of clients and organizations. His children now own and operate the company.

He authored *Knowing and Living Your Purpose©* in 2013, which is available in softcover and PDF at www.ewbp.com and in softcover and Kindle at www.amazon.com. The book covers the breadth and depth of LeRoy's experiences and shows readers the way to know their life's purpose. It is a testimony to 64 years of LeRoy's journey, which led him to uncover his truth and keep returning to living his life with joy and satisfaction through all of life's experiences. It is a series of stories about people transcending their life's struggles. Included are experiences of the work being used to clear away symptoms such as pain, dis-ease, aging, illness, and self-negation.

It is also a teaching book and includes observations, teachings, and methods for doing energy work, woven together with threads of love, joy, and peace, making a tapestry that is whole. The book explains that it does not need to take numerous years of struggle to get back to one's natural state of wellness and vitality.

Both books and LeRoy's website, www.ewbp.com, describe how the Energetic Well Being Process© works. There are also many videos showing how the Process works on www.YouTube.com.

"Our Essentials Workshop was a beautiful experience for all, including me. Everyone went really deep, and there was some significant clearing. Thanks so much for your support and inspiration. All agree this is such a profound energy, and efficient healing system that really works. Much love and gratitude!"

Karuna Joy (Certified EWB Practitioner who is teaching the workshop to others)

"When I describe you to people, I often say you have one of the best personalities I have ever met. I tell them that you embody such self-acceptance that when I stand before you, I fall in love with myself."

Leigh Russell, Certified EWB Practitioner

"LeRoy Malouf is a wonderfully wise energy practitioner. He is not only gifted with the abilities to channel great restorative energies and guidance, but also excellent at teaching you to understand, strengthen, and help yourself. So fasten your seatbelt when LeRoy steps on the pedal. You're in for a wonderfully enlightening ride!"

Daniel Benor, MD, ABIHM, Wholistic Psychotherapist
Author of *Seven Minutes to Natural Pain Release*

Made in the USA
Middletown, DE
09 October 2016